The Complete Practitioners Guide to Take-Home Testing
Tools for Gathering More Valuable Patient Data

Introduction

Accuracy and efficiency are paramount for the health care practitioner in private practice. You are responsible for collecting a large amount of both subjective and objective data in order to establish a "portrait" of your patient in a relatively short period of time. The value of this data is a factor not of the quantity you can accumulate, but rather is a factor of how you utilize the information to achieve your desired outcome.

Take for example a typical scenario in which you gather a comprehensive history from a patient and perhaps baseline laboratory work. A more thorough approach also includes records and interpretive notes from the patient's medical records from other providers. For many practitioners this is well beyond the data-gathering curve before treatment recommendations are made and the information process stops pending results of the medical plan. Most health care providers do not even perform a physical examination as part of their routine data gathering unless there is a particular symptom or risk factor which merits the exam.

From our perspective, all of these methods of data gathering are essential in establishing a good profile of the patient and allow the practitioner to begin their important "detective" work of the patient's case. The difficulty is rarely deciding what treatments to give, but how to identify the underlying causes to specifically treat. The broader the scope of data collected enhances the ability of the practitioner to identify otherwise overlooked clues. Many of the most important clues are not directly associated with the symptom picture your patient presents with, but are representative of areas of dysfunction or imbalance. This more "functional" methodology of data gathering will tremendously enhance your clinical detective skills and make you a more effective practitioner.

The clinical tests discussed in this book are designed to be "take-home" or patient homework exercises. You will find these exercises an invaluable method of gathering additional functional data that will engage your patients and improve treatment compliance. Additionally, a stronger sense of patient accountability is created when you involve them more fully in your data gathering process. We also find that these take home tests serve as a great practice-building tool as frequently a patient will share their take-home tests with others and refer you new patients.

Please visit www.BloodChemistryAnalysis.com to download all the master forms for use within your healthcare practice. We hope that you find the information extremely useful and beneficial to your practice needs.

Dr. Scott Ferguson & Dr. Dicken Weatherby

HCl Challenge Test

Background

The HCl challenge test is designed to help determine the ability of the stomach to produce adequate stomach acid. The body has evolved to release stomach acid in response to appropriate stimuli. Thinking about food, chewing and the presence of certain foods (healthy or not) in the stomach e.g. proteins, milk, calcium salts, coffee… stimulate the release of Gastrin, a hormone secreted by Gastrin cells, or G cells, in the pyloric glands located in the antrum of the stomach[1]. Gastrin strongly stimulates the parietal glands to produce and secrete acid into the stomach. Histamine is another hormone that stimulates acid production. Its effect is potentiated by the presence of Gastrin. Many people have a deficient acid producing process and suffer from hypochlorhydria or in more severe cases achlorhydria.

It is important to remember that stomach acid plays a very important role in human physiology. Some of important functions of stomach acid include:

1. Sterilization of the food we eat

2. Killing ingested parasites, bacteria etc.

3. Allowing for optimal absorption of B12

4. Setting up the pH of the whole GI tract

5. Stimulating duodenal Cholecystokinin and secretin, thus providing the appropriate stimulation for pancreatic secretions to be released

6. Essential for optimum absorption of minerals

Causes of Hypochlorhydria

1. Excessive caffeine, sugar, refined foods, alcohol, chronic overeating, drugs, emotional stress, sympathetic dominant lifestyle

2. Antacid drugs e.g. Tagamet, Pepcid AC, Prilosec, Nexium etc.

3. History of coffee drinking

4. Radical diet changes: Meat to vegetarian, or vegetarian to meat. Veganism

5. Autoimmune disease (antipariteal cell antibody)

Symptoms of Hypochlorhydria

1. Gas, bloating, eructation

2. Food sits and doesn't digest, slow emptying time with a heavy, long lasting, full feeling in the stomach

3. Trouble digesting proteins, may have food sensitivies to proteins

4. Diarrhea/constipation

5. Bloating, gas, heaviness, fullness, worse after eating

---

[1] Guyton, Arthur C, *Textbook of Medical Physiology, 8th ed.*, W.B. Saunders Company, 1991. p. 715

NOTES:

6. Heartburn and indigestion (many use OTC antacids), usually worse when food is in the stomach.

7. Easy satiety, functional dyspepsia; these patients may have constipation, diarrhea or normal stools

8. Many people don't eat in the morning

9. Symptoms worse 1/2-1 hour after meals from eating protein: there's not enough acid to balance the alkali in the duodenum so there's reflux of alkali through the pyloric valve and alkali burns esophageal tissue (not unlike GERDs)

Signs of Hypochlorhydria

1. Joint aches and muscle weakness due to protein maldigestion

2. May have chronic anemia: pallor, bruising, fatigue

3. Nervousness, insomnia

4. Soft, brittle or peeling nails

5. Hair loss in women

6. Telangiectasia of the maxillary area/ Acne Rosacea

Get master copies of all of the handouts in the Take-Home Testing book. Visit:
www.BloodChemistryAnalysis.com

Discussion- Gastric Reflux and Hyper-secretion of Stomach acid

 Many of our patients complain of gastric reflux due to "excess" stomach acid secretion. In our experience hypersecretion of stomach acid is not common. Inappropriate timing of stomach acid however is common, and can produce symptoms in an irritated or inflamed digestive tract.

- For many the reflux of stomach content into the esophagus has more to do with inadequate secretions of stomach acid leading to the putrification of food and the accompanying symptoms of gas, bloating, reflux and belching.

- Antacid therapy may provide temporary relief but does nothing to get to the cure, and are suppressive in the long term.

- One of the best ways to treat this condition is to perform a stomach challenge by taking a small amount of supplemental hydrochloric acid during the middle of a large, complex meal.

- If the dosage does not cause of stomach pain, aggravation or burning, queasiness, abdominal or lower chest discomfort, then slowly increase the dosage over the course of the next few days.

- It is important to proceed as long as the acid supplement is well tolerated.

NOTES:

When would you ask your patient to run this test?

1. To determine whether the patient has sufficient HCl for digestion.

2. To determine the appropriate dose of supplemental stomach acid to use with your patients.

3. To assess for gastric inflammation by challenging the mucosal lining of the stomach.

Supplies you will need to give patients

1. A copy of the handout "HCl Challenge Test" (see handouts section in back of book)

2. 10 HCl capsules or tablets, which are enough to challenge 4 meals.

Directions

- The best meals to challenge are ones that are high in protein and form a substantial complex meal.
- Advise them not to challenge small meals or ones that consist of only fruit, a light salad, or a simple bowl of cereal.
- Meals without protein may cause stomach irritation when challenged with supplemental HCl.

Meal 1: The patient takes 1 capsule of HCl at the **beginning** of the meal, after the first few bites of a substantial complex meal (i.e. one that contains protein). They should note if they experience any mild burning or irritation. If they do, they should stop the challenge and note that they had symptoms after 1 capsule. If they experienced no burning it is appropriate for them to continue. Please see the note below if the stomach irritation is intense.

Meal 2: The patient takes 2 capsules at the **beginning** of the next complex meal, noting any mild burning or irritation. Again, if they experience this the challenge stops at this meal, and they note that 2 capsules produced symptoms on their form. If no symptoms they move on to challenge meal number 3.

Meal 3: The patient takes 3 capsules at the **beginning** of the next complex meal, noting any mild burning or irritation. If no symptoms they proceed onto the last challenge.

Meal 4: This is the last meal to challenge. The patient takes the remaining 4 capsules with their complex meal, noting any mild burning or irritation. If they experience none, they should write no symptoms after 4 capsules on their tracking form.

NOTE: Your patients should stop taking the supplemental HCl if and when they react and have the following symptoms:

1. Feeling of warmth or pressure in your stomach

NOTES:

When would you ask your patients to run this test?

1. To assess your patients eliminative capacity
2. To screen for constipation or diarrhea
3. To screen for changes in your patient's stool. This can provide clues to your patient's gastrointestinal health.

Supplies you will need to give patients

1. A copy of the handout "Bowel Transit Time" (see handouts section in back of book)
2. 8 Charcoal capsules or tablets, which are enough for 2 tests

Directions:

1. The patient swallows 4 charcoal capsules at the evening meal.
2. They should record the date and time that they swallowed the capsules.
3. After every bowel movement, they should observe the stool under bright light.
4. When they first see a black or charcoal gray stool they record the date and time under "Time Color First Appears on the form".
5. They should calculate the number of hours between the time noted under "Time in" and the time noted under "Time Color First Appears" and write this time (in hours) in the form. This is the time it took for the charcoal to pass through the digestive tract.
6. They should continue to examine every stool and note the time and date when the color has completely disappeared.
7. Ideally they should repeat the test by waiting five (5) days to allow the marker to clear fully from the intestines and then repeat the process again, following the same instructions.

Results:

Optimal Bowel Transit Time: 18 – 24 hours

Clinical implications

Clinical Implication	Additional information
Normal Transit Time with Residual color on next stool	This indicates that your patients have an optimal transit time but may be lacking in fiber or water as the charcoal should be expelled in one bowel movement.
Fast Transit Time	A fast transit time is associated with diarrhea, which may be acute or chronic. A fast transit time can be due to a gastrointestinal infection from the following: Parasites (Giardia lamlia, Entamoeba histolytica,

NOTES:

	Cryptosporidium, Isospora), Viral infection (Enterovirus, rotavirus), Bacterial infection (Campylobacter jejuni, Shigella, Salmonella, Yersinia enterocolitica), Intestinal toxins (Clostridium, E. coli, staphylococcus) A fast transit time is associated with a previous antibiotic therapy that has altered the gastrointestinal terrain to such an extent that both digestion and elimination are compromised. A fast transit time may also be due to the use of laxatives or other medications that cause an increased peristalsis within the gastrointestinal tract. One of the main concerns with a chronic fast bowel transit time is malabsorption of key nutrients, both fat and water soluble, and dehydration. Our body has evolved to have the digested food matter spend enough time in the small intestine for optimal absorption of nutrients. A rapid transit time does not allow for this absorption to take place. Other conditions to consider include inflammatory bowel disease, irritable bowel, malabsorption, leaky gut syndrome, emotional stress, food allergies, carbohydrate malabsorption (lactose intolerance), wheat allergy, excess consumption of non-metabolized carbohydrate sweeteners (maltitiol, sorbitol etc.), excess vitamin C intake, insufficient bile output due to gallbladder insufficiency causing fat malabsorption and steatorrhea, and laxative abuse.
Fast Transit Time with Residual color on the next stool	The implications for a fast transit time apply to this type, but this patient probably has a small stool volume hence the residual color on the next stool.
Slow Transit Time	There are organic and functional reasons a patient may present with a slow bowel transit time: **Organic causes** include diverticulitis, fissures, weakness in the rectum or sigmoid colon (often caused by laxative abuse) impaction of fecal material in the bowel, a mass of some kind obstructing the bowel (tumor or pregnancy), inflammation or spasm from pain in the rectum or anal canal. **Functional causes** include a diet that is irritating to the colon, lack of bulk to the stool (fiber absorbs water making the stool soft and allows for enough bulk for the muscles of the large intestine to move the stool through the colon), lack of fluids, insufficient digestion (hypochlorhydria and/or pancreatic insufficiency), stress, hypothyroidism, infection, or even adrenal dysfunction. For some a slow bowel transit time may have a mental/emotional etiology. They may have a neurogenic constipation caused by a repeated voluntary resistance of the urge to have a bowel movement. This can increase in

NOTES:

	situations of increased stress that increases sympathetic outflow, which causes the blood vessels of the colon to constrict (cold, pain, fear etc.)
Slow Transit time with residual color on the next stool	The implications for a slow transit time apply to this type, but this patient not only has a delayed transit time but also a diminished stool volume.

Changes in patient's Stool

Change in Stool	Clinical Implication
Blood on stool	This is always an abnormal state. Blood streaked on outer surface usually indicates hemorrhoids or anal abnormalities; blood present in stool from higher in colon; if transit time is rapid, can be from stomach or duodenum as bright or dark red.
Undigested food	This may indicate insufficient HCL and/or pepsin production. An insufficiently acidic bolus of chyme moving into the intestines may not trigger sufficient pancreatic enzyme production causing pancreatic insufficiency. Also consider that your patient is not chewing their food appropriately.
Mucous on stool	Mucous on the stool is usually due to gastrointestinal irritation (colitis, food sensitivity, pancreatitis). A translucent gelatinous mucus clinging to the surface of formed stool occurs in: spastic constipation; mucous colitis; emotionally disturbed patients; excessive straining at stool.
Loose stool	Loose but not watery stool is associated with mild intestinal irritation and malabsorption.
Hard stool	This is usually due to increased absorption of fluid as a result of prolonged contact of luminal contents with the mucosa of the colon because of delayed transit time (lack of fiber, dehydration, hypochlorhydria).
Floating stool	Consider malabsorption (esp. fats), reduced tract time due to anxiety or irritation, and a high fiber diet. The stool may also be described as slippery or greasy looking.
Ribbon-like shape	**A ribbon-like stool** suggests possibility of spastic bowel, rectal narrowing or stricture (**pencil shaped**), decreased elasticity, or partial obstruction (uterus malposition, prostatitis, polyp, tumor).
Large caliber stool	Consider a high fiber diet or dilation of the viscus of the colon.
Small, round and hard	A condition called scybala this is found with habitual or moderate constipation. Severe fecal retention can produce a large amount of impacted masses in the colon with a small, round and hard stool as overflow.
Brown	A brown colored stool is probably due to Sterobilin (urobilin), a bile pigment derivative resulting from the action of reducing bacteria in bilirubin. It is a normal finding.

NOTES:

Dark brown	A consistently dark brown stool is associated with an excessively alkaline colon that may indicate dysbiosis. A dark brown stool can be a normal finding indicating good bile flow and elimination of fat-soluble toxins.
Yellow	Usually seen with severe diarrhea, may be due to lack of intestinal flora and will also occur from antibiotic use. Consider excessive bile secretions due to over stimulation or irritation to the small intestine.
Black	This is usually a result of bleeding into upper GI tract (ulcer, Crohn's, Colitis, cancer); also the use of drugs, iron, bismuth, charcoal or a heavy meat diet.
Tan or clay colored	This is associated with a blockage of the common bile duct (lack of bile pigments) as well as pancreatic insufficiency, which produces a pale, greasy acholic stool. Consider gall bladder insufficiency or hepatobiliary obstruction.
Offensive odor	Indole and Skatole, intestinal toxins formed from intestinal putrefaction and fermentation by bacteria, are primarily responsible for odor. **Usually offensive odor** – may be due to malabsorption, food decay, dysbiosis **Occasionally offensive-** consider intermittent malabsorption with food decay and dysbiosis.

Related Tests:

Use the following to further assess for gastrointestinal dysfunction:

1. Check the stomach acid reflex point for tenderness. This is located 1 inch below xyphoid and over to the left edge of the rib cage.

2. Check for tenderness in the stomach and upper digestion reflex located in 6th intercostal space on the left

3. Assess the pH of your patient's stomach gastric acid assessment using the Gastrotest (see our book entitled "In-Office Lab Testing- Functional Terrain Analysis" for more details.)

4. Do a functional urinalysis and check for increased urinary indican levels (see our book entitled "In-Office Lab Testing- Functional Terrain Analysis" for more details.)

5. Check for tenderness in the Chapman reflex for the colon located bilaterally along the iliotibial band on the thighs. Palpate the colon for tenderness and tension.

6. Order a chem. screen and check to see whether the protein, globulin, MCV, calcium, iron, and ferritin are in the optimal range. (see our book entitled "Blood Chemistry and CBC Analysis- Clinical Laboratory Testing from a Functional Perspective" for more details.)

7. Order a digestive stool analysis, which will reveal excess undigested meat fibers (can also mean meat allergy, rapid transit time or pancreatic exocrine insufficiency), and a stool pH approaching 7.0 (may also be due to low butyric acid, and/or loss of lactobacillus).

NOTES:

Blood Glucose Monitoring

Background

Our body is constantly monitoring its level of blood glucose and compensates when levels are high or low by releasing various hormones into the blood stream (insulin and glycogen). Unfortunately many people are losing the capacity to self-regulate their own blood sugar levels and are moving down the road of metabolic dysglycemia to diabetes. Many of our patients are unaware that they are losing the ability to regulate their blood sugar levels, and the blood glucose monitoring program is designed to identify whether or not your patients are becoming metabolically dysglycemic.

It is hard for us to help our patients with their blood sugar metabolism issues without knowing how the body regulates blood sugar across the day. Blood glucose levels are affected by a number of factors: exercise, what you eat, when you ate, what medications you are on etc. The blood glucose monitoring handout (see handouts section in back of book), which measures blood glucose levels across the day, is the key process of developing a blood glucose profile on your patients.

Discussion

The blood glucose profile will tell you how your patient's lifestyle and diet affect their blood sugar levels. Blood glucose data, along with information about meals, exercise, medications etc. are recorded onto a convenient patient handout, which the patient fills in and brings back to the office for interpretation.

How often should you ask your patients to perform a blood sugar profile?

Depending on the severity of their blood sugar dysregulation it may be necessary to ask your patients to do this profile periodically while you change their treatment plan to normalize their blood glucose levels.

What kind of blood glucose measuring system should be used?

We highly recommend using a hand-held electronic blood glucose measuring device called a glucometer. The meter is used with disposable strips that collect a drop of blood from your patient's finger. The meter reads the amount of glucose in that drop of blood and displays a numerical reading on the display screen. We recommend that your clinic purchases one or more of these devices and either lends or rents them out to the patients for their own use. The device we recommend is the Elite Meter from Bayer, either the XL or the standard. This recommendation comes from Richard Bernstein, MD, a pioneer and leader in the field of Diabetes and author of "Dr. Bernstein's Diabetes Solution". If you are working with diabetic patients we highly recommend this book.[2]

---

[2] Bernstein, Richard, *Dr. Bernstein's Diabetes Solution,*, Little, Brown, 1997.

NOTES:

When would you ask your patients to run this test?

1. To screen for potential blood sugar dysregulation problems
2. To monitor the effects of dietary changes on blood sugar levels

Supplies you will need to give patients

1. A copy of the handouts "Directions for Measuring Blood Glucose" and "Blood Sugar Tracking Form" (see handouts section in back of book)
2. Glucometer, lancets, spring-loaded finger stick device, test strips.

Directions:

Techniques for measuring blood glucose.[3]

1. Instruct patients to wash their hands. Invisible material on the fingers can cause erroneous readings.
2. Do not wipe fingers with alcohol. This only dries the finger out and can cause calluses. It is highly unlikely that you will get a finger infection by not using alcohol.
3. Rinse the fingers under warm water unless the fingers are already warm. Blood flow increases when the fingers are warm.
4. Sort out the supplies for measuring blood glucose: finger-stick device loaded with a sterile lancet, the glucometer, test strips, and tissue for blotting the blood.
5. Insert a fresh strip into the glucometer. Follow the directions for loading the test strips into your particular unit.
6. The spring loaded finger-stick device is used to obtain a drop of blood. The pressure of the device on the finger determines how deep the lancet will puncture the skin. It should be deep enough to get an adequate amount of blood, but not so deep as to cause bruising or pain.
7. Contrary to popular opinion one of the best areas for getting a blood sample is the back of the hand. Prick the fingers near the nails, or between the first and second joints. The advantages of using these areas are less pain and more chance of getting an adequate drop of blood. You will also prevent calluses by repeatedly using the fleshy pads on the finger tips. By all means use these areas too if the thought of pricking the back of hand is off-putting.
8. Cock the spring-loaded finger stick device and prick any finger. Squeeze the finger using a pumping action rather than constant pressure. You should aim to get a drop of blood about 1/16th of an inch in diameter.
9. Touch the blood to the test strip.
10. The glucometer will start a count down procedure once the blood has been absorbed by the test strip. After the countdown has started inspect the drop of blood to see that the test strip has been properly covered by the blood drop. If not discard the strip and begin the process over again. It is essential that the strip be covered in blood to prevent erroneous readings.

---

[3] Bernstein, Richard, *Dr. Bernstein's Diabetes Solution,*, Little, Brown, 1997. p.70 – 71

NOTES:

11. If you are the only person using the glucometer it is not necessary to use a fresh lancet every time. If others are using the unit, please remove the used lancet to prevent possible contamination for future users.
12. The whole process from start to finish should take approximately 2 minutes.
13. Record the number from the glucometer on your form.

Results and Interpretation

For most non-diabetic individuals the optimal blood glucose level should be between 80 and 100 mg/dl. Ideally you should aim to keep your patients blood glucose levels as close to 90 mg/dl as possible. This reflects optimal physiological control of blood glucose.

Unless your patient had an excessively sweet meal i.e. dessert or refined carbohydrates their blood sugar an hour after a meal should have returned into the optimal range. If your patient's readings are moving back and forth across the day between 70 and 130 mg/dl they are caught on the blood sugar roller coaster and need to be on a treatment plan that will help stabilize the roller coaster nature of their blood glucose swings.

Related Tests:

Use the following to further assess for blood sugar dysregulation:

1. Check for tenderness in the Chapman reflex for the liver-gallbladder located over the 6th intercostal space on the right.
2. Check for tenderness in the Liver point located on the 3rd rib, 3" to the right of the sternum, at the costochondral junction.
3. Check for tenderness underneath the right rib cage.
4. Check for tenderness or nodularity in the right thenar pad, which is a pancreas indicator if tender.
5. Check for tenderness or guarding at the head of the pancreas located in the upper left quadrant of the abdominal region 1/2 to 2/3 of the way between the umbilicus and the angel of the ribs.
6. Run a six hour glucose-insulin tolerance test.

Also consider checking for low functioning adrenal glands:

1. Check for tenderness in the inguinal ligament bilaterally.
2. Check for tenderness at the medial knee bilaterally, at the insertion of the sartorius muscle at the Pes Anserine.
3. Check for a paradoxical pupillary reflex by shining a light into a patient's eye and grading the reaction of the pupil. A pupil that fails to constrict indicates adrenal exhaustion.
4. Check for the presence of postural hypotension. A drop of more than 10 points is an indication of adrenal insufficiency.
5. Check for a chronic short leg due to a posterior-inferior ilium.

NOTES:

Zinc Taste Test

Background

Zinc is one of the most important trace minerals. Its effects on the body are far-reaching due to its role in more enzyme systems than the rest of all the trace minerals combined. Zinc is a major component of over 70 metalloenzyme complexes, which catalyze major biochemical reactions in the body. One of the most important of these is carbonic anhydrase, the enzyme that catalyzes the carbonic acid-bicarbonate buffering system, without which we would not survive. It is also essential in the maintenance of our basal metabolic rate and zinc deficiency has been associated with a decreased Basal Metabolic Rate (BMR).

Despite its essentiality in life processes, no functional store of zinc appears to exist. Most of the body's zinc is locked away in bone and protein, which is one of the reasons that zinc deficiency is very common. Zinc deficiency is also caused by impaired absorption, due to hypochlorhydria, inhibition by certain nutrients (iron), and drugs (birth control pills and steroids), and a lack of zinc in the soil.

Zinc deficiency has a large impact on cellular function and metabolism. Zinc deficiency is associated with a loss of taste and smell, reduced immunity, failure to thrive, reproductive difficulties, especially in men, loss of appetite, and various skin disorders including, seborrhea, scaling or flaking skin, and acne.

Discussion

Zinc deficiency can lead to unnecessary suffering, making the Zinc Taste test a valuable assessment for most patients. The test is a non-invasive method of determining a patient's physiological zinc status. It is a functional assessment as opposed to the quantitative assessment for zinc, such as serum or plasma zinc studies.

- Zinc deficiency is strongly associated with a loss of taste acuity and this lack of "gustatory sensitivity" has been shown to be a possible indication of the "functional" availability of zinc.

- A percentage of patients presenting with functional zinc deficiency are also deficient in vitamin B6 and magnesium, synergistic nutrients with zinc. If a patient fails the ZTT and does not respond to zinc therapy, they should be evaluated for B6 and magnesium status to find out the cause of the problem.

- An initial short course of liquid zinc therapy is clinically more useful than tableted zinc, due to the fact that HCl production is also zinc dependent and tableted zinc may not be absorbed due to hypochlorhydria.

NOTES:

When would you ask your patients to run this test?

1. A non-invasive, quick and in-expensive method to assess their zinc status.
2. If a deficiency is noted, this test can determine how deficient they are.

Supplies you will need to give patients

1. A copy of the handouts "Zinc Taste Test" and "Zinc Challenge Tracking Form" (see handouts section in back of book).
2. 1 bottle of aqueous zinc (zinc sulphate), which is enough to perform a full zinc challenge test.

Directions:

This test is done in two parts. The first part is to determine whether or not a zinc deficiency is present. The second part involves a zinc challenge, which uses the same test to determine how zinc deficient they are.

Basic test instructions:

1. Patient's mouth should be free of any strong tastes
2. Patient holds and swishes ¼ ounce of aqueous zinc in their mouth
3. Start timing and have patient indicate when they first taste the solution
4. Have them swallow after 15 seconds
5. Ask them to describe the strength of taste or presence of an after taste
6. Record strength of taste and seconds it took to taste the solution

Ranges:

Level	Interpretation	Description
1	**Optimal Zinc levels**	An immediate, unpleasant and obviously adverse taste in a few seconds (strongly metallic)
2	**Mild zinc deficiency**	A definite but not strongly unpleasant taste is noted in 4-6 seconds and tends to intensify with time. (delayed metallic)
3	**Moderate Zinc Deficient**	No taste noted initially, but develops in 7-13 seconds. May be described as sweet or bitter
4	**Very Zinc Deficient**	Tasteless or "tastes like water".

Clinical implications

Levels 3 or 4 represent a zinc deficiency and should be treated by following the following zinc challenge protocol. (Please see next page for details)

NOTES:

Zinc Challenge

Discussion

The zinc challenge is used to assess how zinc deficient your patient may be and how much zinc therapy is needed.

- The zinc challenge uses repeated challenges with the aqueous zinc to determine how much aqueous zinc is needed to begin supplementation.

- Aqueous zinc can be used therapeutically in the initial stages of zinc supplementation. Although low dose, it is an optimal form to enhance zinc absorption. It is much less dependent on optimal hydrochloric acid levels than other forms of zinc.

Supplies you will need to give patients

1. A copy of the handouts "Zinc Taste Test" and "Zinc Challenge Tracking Form" (see handouts section in back of book).

2. 1 bottle of aqueous zinc, which is enough to perform a full zinc challenge test.

Zinc Challenge Directions

1. Begin with standard the Zinc Taste test as previously described

2. Repeat the process successively, resting 30 seconds between tests, and noting changes in strength of taste

3. Note how many challenges it takes for the patient to reach a strong metallic taste indicating zinc saturation

Clinical implications

- We can approximate that the number of challenges will equal the number of bottles of aqueous zinc that the patient needs to begin a zinc maintenance program.

- Dosage for aqueous zinc supplementation is 1 ounce 2X/day with meals

- After the course of aqueous zinc begin supplementation with 45 mg of zinc 2 times a day for 60 days. At this time redo the ZTT.

What if the patient is unable to reach a metallic taste with the zinc challenge?

Consider the following options:

1. Treat presumptively if zinc deficiency signs are present.

2. Screen with white blood cell zinc and magnesium levels (a synergistic nutrient with zinc).

NOTES:

3. Rule out Vitamin B6 deficiency with serum homocysteine.

4. If indicated start treating with B6 and Magnesium.

5. Consider damaged olfactory centers, which compromise the ability to taste and smell (trauma, smoking).

Note: Zinc is best taken with meals to prevent nausea, which is most often seen in people who are both zinc deficient and hypochlorhydric.

Interfering Factors:

Vitamin B6 or Magnesium deficiency can cause a false positive result.

Related Tests:

Use the following to further assess for other mineral deficiencies

1. Assess for mineral deficiency using Tissue Mineral Assessment test. Place a standard blood pressure cuff around the largest portion of the patient's calf muscle (sitting). Instruct the patient to let you know when they feel the onset of cramping pain and gradually inflate the cuff. Stop and deflate immediately when threshold has been reached. Less than 200 mmHg is considered deficient in minerals. Use the neurolingual testing to challenge the body with several different types of minerals and other co-factors to see which combination of minerals and co-factors increases the threshold above 200mmHg.

2. Assess for mineral insufficiency by using Dr. Kane's mineral assessment tests.

3. Assess the impact of mineral deficiencies on the body's acid buffering capacities by using Dr. Bieler's salivary pH acid challenge.

Please see our book entitled "In-Office Lab Testing- Functional Terrain Analysis" for more details on these tests.

NOTES:

Basal Body Temperature Test

Background

- The thyroid hormones, thyroxine (T4) and Triiodothyronine (T3) play a large role in maintaining metabolic activity. T3 is the most potent form of thyroid hormone and has the strongest effect on the metabolic rate. Under the influence of T3 the mitochondria in the cells will increase, thus increasing the metabolic activity of the cell. T3, along with the catecholamine hormones from the adrenal glands, also stimulates oxygen utilization and increases energy turnover, which will increase heat production.[4] A reduced core body temperature is one of the hallmarks of thyroid hormone deficiency and hypothyroidism.

- There is considerable evidence that blood tests often fail to detect hypothyroidism. It appears that many individuals have "tissue resistance" to thyroid hormone, analogous to insulin resistance. For this reason it is useful to have other means of detecting an under-active thyroid gland, and the basal body temperature test is a means to do this.

Discussion

The basal body temperature test is designed to measure the core body temperature over time. It assesses both axillary and oral temperature across the day to give a complete picture of all the controlling factors that contribute to basal metabolism.

- A low axillary temperature first thing in the morning is suggestive of hypothyroidism. The axillary temperature is used because it closely correlates with thyroid function.

- Oral temperatures, taken across the day, help assess the adrenal contribution to basal metabolism and can indicate blood sugar swings, particularly if the before and after lunch temperatures are significantly different.

- Axillary and oral temperatures are taken for two days and compared to verify the absence of oral lesions that may cause an elevated oral temperature unrelated to basal metabolic status.

- It has been suggested that a lowered basal body temperature may be due to a deficiency of essential trace minerals (zinc, copper, and selenium) rather than a deficiency of thyroid hormone.[5] These minerals are essential for the peripheral conversion of T4 into T3.

When would you ask your patients to run this test?

---

[4] Despopoulos, Agamemnon. *Color Atlas of Physiology, 4th Ed.* Thieme Medical Publishers, Inc., New York, 1991. p252

[5] Passwater, Richard A., Ph.D. Trace Elements, Hair analysis and Nutrition. Keats Publishing, Inc. New Canaan, CT. 1983. p172.

NOTES:

1. To assess the hormonal influences on metabolism
2. To help identify sub-clinical hypothyroidism
3. To identify adrenal and blood sugar influences on basal metabolism

When to take the test

For pre-menopausal women

- The temperature should be taken starting the second day of menstruation. This is because a temperature rise occurs around the time of ovulation, which may lead to incorrect interpretation of the test.

- If they miss a day, that is OK, but they should be sure to finish the testing before ovulation.

For men, and for women who are menopausal or post-menopausal

- It makes no difference when the temperatures are taken. However, they should not do the test if they have an infection or any other condition that would raise their temperature.

Supplies you will need to give patients

1. A copy of the handout "Basal Body Temperature Test" (see handouts section in back of book).
2. A basal body thermometer.

Directions:

1. Your patients should use either a mercury thermometer (a basal body thermometer is more accurate), or a good quality digital thermometer. They will need to shake down the mercury thermometer down the night before to 96 degrees or less and put it by the bedside.

2. In the morning, as soon as they wake up, they put the thermometer deep in their armpit for ten minutes and record the temperature to 1/10 of a degree. They need to do this before getting out of bed, having anything to eat or drink, or engaging in any activity. This will measure their lowest temperature of the day, which correlates with thyroid gland function.

3. All of the temperature readings are recorded on the Basal Body Temperature Handout.

4. Have them record their axillary temperature for 2 days and then average it out.

5. Next shake the thermometer down and immediately take an oral temperature for 3 minutes. They record this temperature as "a.m. by mouth" for 7 days.

6. Repeat the oral temperature at three hour intervals for 7 days.

NOTES:

7. Record the time when meals are consumed. They should make note of the foods eaten on back of the handout. This can help determine foods that may be causing blood sugar swings.

8. Note when activity has changed (i.e. I went for a walk).

9. They bring the form filled out and your office should work out the averages.

10. The next page has a handout with directions for doing the test and a chart for filling out the results.

Optimal Results

The normal axillary temperature should ideally be 97.8°-98.2°F

The normal oral temperature should ideally be 98.6°F

Axillary and oral temperatures should be within 1°F of each other

Clinical Interpretation

Low average axillary temperature

Clinical Result	Interpretation
If the average first morning axillary temperature is below 97.6°	Suspect hypothyroidism and low basal metabolism. Evaluate this with other clinical findings for hypothyroidism.

Low average oral temperature

Clinical Result	Interpretation
If the average oral temperature is below 98.4°	Suspect hypothyroidism and low basal metabolic activity. Evaluate this with other clinical findings for hypothyroidism.

Oral temperature fluctuations across the day

Clinical Result	Interpretation
Oral temperature fluctuations across the day	When activity levels are constant, variations in oral temperature throughout the day may indicate blood sugar swings, especially if the before and after lunch temperatures are significantly different (i.e. low prior to lunch and higher after lunch, often ½ to 1½ degree variation)

19

NOTES:

Interfering factors

1. Menstruation
2. Excess movement before taking the axillary temperature
3. Use of an electric blanket, hot water bottles
4. Fever
5. Some type of inflammation: earache, toothache, oral lesions etc.
6. Medications: birth control pills, cortisone, prednisone, DHEA, progesterone, estrogen

Further Assessment

Use the following tests to further assess low thyroid function

1. Check for tenderness in the Chapman reflex for the thyroid located in the right second intercostal space near the sternum
2. Check for a delayed Achilles return reflex, which is a strong sign of a hypo-functioning thyroid
3. Check for general costochondral tenderness, a thyroid indicator
4. Check for pre-tibial edema, a sign of a hypo-functioning thyroid
5. Iodine patch test: Use a tincture of 2% iodine solution, and paint a 3" by 3" square on the patient's abdomen. The patient is to leave the patch unwashed until it disappears. The square should still be there in 24 hours. If it has disappeared, there is an indication of iodine need
6. Run a blood chemistry thyroid panel and look for changes in TSH, T4, T3, FTI and T3-Uptake (see our book entitled "Blood Chemistry and CBC Analysis- Clinical Laboratory Testing from a Functional Perspective" for more details.)

NOTES:

Iodine Patch Test

Background

Iodine is a nutrient that is deficient in many people. It has been associated with goiter, an enlargement of the neck seen in many individuals living in iodine deficient areas. In the 1900s the area around the Great Lakes was known as the "goiter belt" due to the iodine deficient soil and the prevalence of goiter in the population. The connection between iodine and goiter is the thyroid gland. Iodine is essential for thyroid function, being an integral part of thyroxine (T4) and Triiodothyronine (T3) molecules. Iodine deficiency can cause an increase in the number and size of the epithelial cells of the thyroid gland itself.[6]

The majority of the body's iodine, about 20 to 30 mg in the average adult body, is stored in the thyroid in the form of thyroid hormone. Less than 1mg is found in the blood, and trace amounts are found in the tissue. Iodine supplementation in the past was administered by painting iodine onto the skin in a transdermal application. This forms the basis for the iodine patch test.

Symptoms of iodine deficiency[7]

1. Lowered vitality
2. Inability to think clearly
3. Low resistance to infection
4. Teeth defects and deformities
5. Obesity
6. Cretinism
7. Circulatory disorders
8. Abnormal breast tissue growth

Discussion

 The iodine patch test is a functional assessment for iodine status in the body. By painting the skin with a 2% solution of iodine we can see how quickly the body absorbs the available iodine.

- If there is a deficiency or need for iodine the slightly brownish yellow stain will fade in less than 24 hours.

- This indicates that there is not sufficient enough iodine to normalize thyroid secretions.

- The quicker the iodine fades, the greater the deficiency can be assumed to be.

---

[6] Passwater, Richard A., Ph.D. Trace Elements, Hair analysis and Nutrition. Keats Publishing, Inc. New Canaan, CT. 1983. p171.
[7] Ibid

NOTES:

Functions of Iodine

1. Principal role in the manufacturer of thyroid hormone

2. Modulation of the effect of estrogen on breast tissue. Dr. Eskin, a gynecological endocrinologist, has shown that estrogen hastens the development of breast dysplasia in women who are iodine deficient.[8]

3. The conversion of estrone and estradiol into estriol

When would you ask your patients to run this test?

1. When iodine deficiency is suspected

2. Patients present with signs of hypothyroidism

3. Patients with low basal body temperatures

Supplies you will need to give patients

1. A copy of the handout "Iodine Patch Test"

2. 1 bottle of topical 2% iodine solution.

Directions:

1. Your patient will paint their skin with a 2 inch square patch of 2% iodine solution.

2. They should avoid soaking in hot tubs or baths for 24 hours, as the chlorine or bromine in the water will cause the iodine to patch to come off.

3. They should note how soon after application the iodine patch has disappeared.

Get master copies of all of the handouts in the Take-Home Testing book. Visit:
www.BloodChemistryAnalysis.com

Results:

Color lasts for > 24 hours	Sufficient iodine
Color fades in < 24 hours	Deficient iodine

---

[8] Passwater, Richard A., Ph.D. Trace Elements, Hair analysis and Nutrition. Keats Publishing, Inc. New Canaan, CT. 1983. p173.

NOTES:

Clinical implications

As was mentioned above, the quicker the iodine fades, the greater the deficiency can be assumed to be. The following protocol should be implemented until sufficiency is obtained i.e. the stain remains for a minimum of 24 hours:

20-30 drops of liquid iodine (as potassium iodide) per day

Interfering Factors:

Patients may react to the topical application of iodine or they may present with symptoms of iodism (too much iodine) during iodine supplementation. The symptoms of iodism are tachycardia, skin irritation, thinning of secretions (watery eyes, nose, saliva), nervousness and headache.

Related Tests:

Use the following tests to further assess low thyroid function

1. Check for tenderness in the Chapman reflex for the thyroid located in the right second intercostal space near the sternum
2. Check for a delayed Achilles return reflex, which is a strong sign of a hypo-functioning thyroid
3. Check for general costochondral tenderness and pre-tibial edema, a sign of a hypo-functioning thyroid
4. Run a blood chemistry thyroid panel and look for changes in TSH, T4, T3, FTI and T3-Uptake (see our book entitled "Blood Chemistry and CBC Analysis-Clinical Laboratory Testing from a Functional Perspective" for more details.)

NOTES:

Metabolic pH Assessment

Background

The terms acidosis and alkalosis are often used indiscriminately. Acidosis, for instance, is blamed for many of the ills of modern living. These claims are made without a true appreciation for biochemistry and physiology of pH regulation in the body. The following section details a number of simple tests that can be used to determine whether or not your patient has an imbalance in acid-alkaline regulation. It is important to remember that we are talking about functional imbalances in the acid/alkaline system, and not the pathological variances in pH that are often seen in the emergency room.

Why is it important to uncover an acid/alkaline imbalance in my patients?

A balanced internal pH is essential for many of the homeostatic mechanisms in the body to work. We are all aware of the need for acidity in the stomach and alkalinity in the small intestine to ensure optimal digestion. Many other systems of the body also operate most effectively with a properly balanced pH. The following is a list of some of the problems that can occur if the pH is out of balance:

1. **Enzyme systems in the body fail to work**. There are thousands of enzyme reactions taking place in our bodies every second. Each of these reactions is like a complex key that needs to "fit" into a specific keyhole. If blood pH is off balance even a little, some important keys are not "fitting" their respective slots. Enzyme function and the essential chemical reactions they facilitate begin to suffer.

2. **The oxygen delivery mechanisms in the blood become compromised**. The body stores excess acidity in the extracellular matrix (the spaces around the cells) of the tissues. The blood, in order to compensate for this, becomes increasingly alkaline. With rising alkalinity, the red blood cells can saturate themselves in oxygen. Increasing oxygen saturation seems like a good thing, until you realize that the major problem is the red blood cells cannot release the oxygen. If the blood cells cannot let go of the oxygen, then the oxygen isn't getting into the cells of the body leading to tissue hypoxia and decreased production of ATP. It is becoming clearer from research that low oxygen delivery to cells is a major factor in most, if not all, degenerative conditions, and it is well known that cancer grows in an oxygen deficient environment.

3. **Blood sugar dysregulation:** Insulin facilitates the movement of glucose into the cell. The ability of the cells to recognize insulin is greatly affected by pH fluctuations in the blood. The brain is one organ that is especially vulnerable to this phenomenon because it cannot store glucose and as such relies on the second to second supply of glucose from the bloodstream. pH fluctuations in the blood are perhaps one of the reasons for much of the blood sugar dysregulation seen today.

NOTES:

4. **Digestive function becomes compromised.** Pancreatic insufficiency is influenced by the body using alkaline pancreatic juices to buffer an acidic blood. Hypochlorhydria is influenced by the body using acidic stomach secretions to buffer an alkaline blood.

5. **Electrolyte and mineral imbalance.** A catch-22 situation occurs in the body when the pH of the blood begins to drift. As we have seen above the body uses alkaline minerals and digestive juices to buffer the blood. Unfortunately the use of the digestive juices to buffer the blood leads to less than optimal digestion, which has a profound effect on the digestion, absorption and assimilation of the alkaline minerals that the body uses to buffer the blood! The availability of these essential electrolytes and minerals is compromised, causing an electrolyte and mineral imbalance. Acids bind up the minerals in the buffering system and they are no longer available to act as the co-factors for the thousands of mineral dependent enzyme reactions. An electrolyte imbalance will have an effect on the ability of both the extracellular fluid to carry nutrients and waste in and out of the cell, and the cell to carry on oxidation and other essential metabolic processes.

6. **The electrical potential of the cell begins to change.** pH imbalances in the extracellular fluids interferes with the potential energy of the cell. The electrical cell potential is usually between –70 to -90mV, which is the optimal range for the movement of nutrients into the cell and waste products out of the cell. Hyperacidity, heavy metals in the extracellular matrix and possibly electromagnetic stress from microwaves and cellular phones drop the voltage as low as 0mV. Under these circumstances, the cells are no longer able to remove waste. Instead they store waste, which greatly reduces their function. As cellular function becomes compromised so does the production of ATP.

How does the body maintain optimal pH?

- The body uses a number of complex buffering systems to keep pH within a normal and optimal range.

1° Buffering System	2° Buffering Systems
1. Bicarbonate buffering system (lungs and kidneys)	1. Alkaline minerals 2. Urea cycle (liver) and ammonia 3. Digestive system
The system used for about 90% of acid/alkaline buffering	The systems used for about 10% of acid/alkaline buffering

1° Buffering – the Bicarbonate Buffering System

The bicarbonate buffering system is the primary extracellular buffering system of the body. It accounts for about 90% of the body's extracellular pH buffering. In this system, carbon dioxide, an acidic by-product of oxidative phosphorylation, combines with water using an enzyme called carbonic anhydrase, (an enzyme that needs the mineral zinc as a co-enzyme), to form carbonic acid. Carbonic acid is fairly unstable in solution and will dissociate into its ionic form of a bicarbonate ion and a hydrogen ion.

NOTES:

The body regulates the primary buffering system using two mechanisms of control:

1. **Respiratory system**

   a. By altering the respiration rate and depth of breathing the body can change the relative concentration of CO_2 in the blood and therefore control pH fluctuations.

   b. By increasing the respiration rate i.e. through hyperventilation, more CO_2 is expelled from the body, which in turn raises the pH (more alkaline)

   c. By decreasing the respiration rate i.e. through hypoventilation, less CO_2 is expelled from the body, which lowers the pH (more acidic)

2. **The Kidney**

   a. By altering the kidney's ability to reabsorb or excrete bicarbonate and H^+ the body can change the relative concentration of bicarbonate or H+ in the blood.

   b. Increased reabsorption of bicarbonate by the kidney in the descending loop of Henle will increase blood bicarbonate and thus raise the pH (more alkaline)

   c. Decreased reabsorption or increased excretion of bicarbonate will decrease blood bicarbonate and thus lower the pH (more acidic)

What happens when these mechanisms are compromised?

There are four main patterns of acid/alkaline imbalance that are seen when factors outside of the body's control begin to alter the body's pH this happens:

1. **Metabolic acidosis** 2. **Metabolic alkalosis**	3. **Respiratory acidosis** 4. **Respiratory Alkalosis**
• Two patterns of acid/base imbalance that are caused by alterations in bicarbonate (HCO_3^-) or H+ concentrations	• Two patterns of acid/base imbalance caused by alterations in CO_2 concentrations

In these situations, the bicarbonate buffer begins to compensate:

1. The body begins to alter the respiration rate and depth of breathing in order to compensate by lowering or raising the amount of dissolved CO^2.

2. The body begins to alter the reabsorption or excretion of either bicarbonate ($HCO3^-$) or H+ via the renal tubules.

Clinical determination of patterns of acid/alkaline imbalance

When we are making a clinical determination of an acid/alkaline imbalance, we are measuring the body's compensatory mechanisms at work. It is important to remember the following:

NOTES:

1. Acid/alkaline imbalances in the bicarbonate buffering system **always** involve the respiratory functions

2. Acid/alkaline imbalances in the bicarbonate buffering system **always** involve the kidneys.

It is also important to remember to ask yourself whether you are looking at the primary cause of the problem or the body's defense or compensation. This is most easily seen in the respiratory system, which is always associated with an acidosis or alkalosis.

The respiratory system can be the primary cause of the imbalance, or, it can be the primary defense in compensation for the imbalance. Whether as cause or an effect, the respiratory system is always part of the clinical picture in evaluating the patterns of acid/alkaline imbalance in the bicarbonate buffering system.

Respiratory system as a 1° cause of acid/alkaline imbalance		Respiratory system as a compensation for acid/alkaline imbalance	
• Causative in Respiratory acidosis and Respiratory alkalosis		• Compensatory in Metabolic acidosis and Metabolic alkalosis	
Respiratory acidosis	• Caused by hypoventilation • CO_2 produced faster than it can be blown off • ↑ carbonic acid retention → acidosis	**Metabolic acidosis**	• Respiratory activity is increased • CO_2 blown off to lower carbonic acid levels
Respiratory alkalosis	• Caused by hyperventilation • CO_2 blown off faster than it can be produced • ↓ carbonic acid levels→ alkalosis.	**Metabolic alkalosis**	• Respiratory activity slowed down • Retention of CO_2 in the form of carbonic acid to decrease the alkalosis.

NOTES:

Clinical assessment of acid/alkaline imbalances

The clinical assessment of acid-alkaline imbalances is best observed by looking at the patterns between the following:

1. Breath holding time
2. Respiration rate
3. Urine pH
4. Saliva pH

Breath holding time and respiration rate

Breath holding time and respiration rate are used to measure the involvement of the respiratory system in patterns of acid/alkaline imbalance in the bicarbonate buffering system.

Since the respiratory system accounts for 50%-70% of pH compensation, the breath holding time and the respiration rate are the main tests used to indicate the **presence** of an acidosis or alkalosis.

NOTE: If your patient has a normal breath hold time and respiration rate then there is *no* imbalance in the primary buffering system

Urine pH and Salivary pH

The urine pH and salivary pH are used to help identify the **type** of acidosis or alkalosis, but not the presence of acidosis or alkalosis—only the breath hold time and respiration do that.

The following section will go into more detail on the specific tests.

NOTES:

Breath – Hold Test

Discussion

 In the absence of cardiovascular, pulmonary or respiratory tract infections, breath-holding time reflects acid/alkaline imbalance.

- In an acidosis there is a decreased transport and uptake of oxygen by the body, which leads to a decreased breath holding time.

- In an alkalosis there is a slight increased uptake and transport of oxygen, as well as a compensatory suppression of the respiratory center, which leads to the ability to hold one's breath longer.

When would you ask your patient to run this test?

1. To check for the presence of an acid/alkaline imbalance

Directions

This test is an actual measurement of how long the patient can hold a deep breath. It is hard to time ones own breath-hold time, so it is best to ask your patients to have a family member or friend do the timing. The patient should be seated and should take a deep breath and hold it as long as they can. A stopwatch or timer can be used to time the breath holding. When the patient can no longer hold their breath they should let it out, and the seconds the breath was held should be recorded on the handout (see handouts section in back of book).

. **Results:**
   Normal: 40-65 seconds

Clinical implications

INCREASED BREATH-HOLD TIME

Clinical Implication	Additional information
Metabolic alkalosis Respiratory alkalosis	Alkalosis causes an increased oxygen uptake and transport leading to an increased ability to hold ones breath

DECREASED BREATH-HOLD TIME

Clinical Implication	Additional information
Metabolic acidosis Respiratory acidosis	In acidosis a decreased transport and uptake of oxygen by the body leads to a decreased breath holding time.
Anemia	Decreased oxygen-carrying capacity of red-blood cells due to anemia may decrease breath-hold time
Other causes include:	Antioxidant deficiency, emotional stress, anxiety

NOTES:

Respiratory Rate

Discussion

 Respiratory rate is used in determining acid/alkaline imbalances in your patients. The respiratory rate is set from the respiratory centers in the brain and responds to oxygen saturation of blood that flows through the aortic and carotid arteries.

When would you ask your patients to run this test?

1. To check for an acid/alkaline imbalance

Supplies you will need to give patients

1. A copy of the handout "Metabolic pH Assessment Form" (see handouts section in back of book).

Directions

This test is a measurement of respiratory rate. It is best not to have your patients measure their own respiratory rate because they will invariably alter their breathing rate and skew the results. Ask them to have a friend or family member count the number of breaths in a full minute. Using a stopwatch, a timer or a watch with a second-hand they can either watch the rise and fall of the chest, or place a hand on the abdomen and count the number of breaths in a full minute. Remember to tell them to count one full cycle of inhalation and exhalation as one breath.

Results:

Normal: 14 – 18 respiratory cycles/minute

Clinical implications

INCREASED RESPIRATORY RATE

Clinical Implication	Additional information
Metabolic acidosis	In metabolic acidosis the body increases respiratory rate as a means of blowing off CO_2 and thus lowering carbonic acid levels to relieve the acidosis.
Respiratory acidosis (compensation)	The increased respiratory rate is a sign of compensation by the body in dealing with respiratory acidosis, which has an etiology in hypoventilation i.e. CO_2 levels increase because the body is unable to blow it off (e.g. in asthma and emphysema). The increased respiration rate is the body's way of compensating. The breathing is rapid and often shallow.
Respiratory alkalosis (Primary cause/acute)	Respiratory alkalosis is caused by hyperventilation or an increased respiratory rate. In the acute or primary phase there is hyperventilation, as the body begins to compensate we see the respiration rate decrease.

NOTES:

Acidic urine- Urine pH < 6.4

Acidic urine indicates an abundance of exogenously or endogenously produced acids, which are being excreted by the kidney.

Clinical Implication	Additional information
Acidosis (respiratory and metabolic)	The body responds to an acidosis by causing the kidneys to dump hydrogen and ammonia thus creating acidic urine.
Carbohydrate and fat maldigestion	People who are consistently acidic (below 6.4 pH) do not optimally digest carbohydrates and fats.

NOTES:

Salivary pH

Discussion

Salivary pH is influenced by a number of different physiological buffering mechanisms that work to keep the salivary pH within an optimum range for digestion.

- The buffering system that has the largest single effect on salivary pH is the relative concentration of free CO_2 and combined CO_2, in the form of carbonic acid (H_2CO_3).
  a. A high CO_2 concentration in the blood will cause an increase in carbonic acid, which will cause acidic saliva. This pattern is seen in respiratory acidosis and metabolic alkalosis.
  b. A low CO_2 concentration will cause a decrease in carbonic acid, which in turn will lead to alkaline saliva. This pattern is seen in respiratory alkalosis and metabolic acidosis.
- Salivary pH should have a slightly alkaline reading of 7.1 -7.4. This alkalinity in the saliva provides the correct pH for optimum amylase activity. When there are enough reserves to buffer the acid produced naturally by cellular activity, saliva pH will register around 7.1-7.4. Readings of considerably lower or higher than this usually indicate that the body has alkaline mineral deficiencies and food will not be assimilated very well due to inefficient digestive enzyme activity.

Supplies you will need to give patients

1. A copy of the handout "Metabolic pH Assessment Form" (see handouts section in back of book).
2. 1 roll of pH paper

Directions:

Testing must be done at least 30 minutes from any food or beverage. The patient places a pH testing strip in their mouth on top of the tongue. They should get it good and moist. Remember to tell them that the lips must remain closed, as clinical readings of salivary pH must not allow exposure of the sample to air, which can result in inaccurate readings. Immediately after removing the pH strip (reading must be made within 3 seconds) they compare the strip with the color code on the box.

When would you ask your patient to run this test?

1. To assess their acid/alkaline balance
2. As a good general indicator for carbohydrate digestion
3. As a good assessment for Essential Fatty Acid (EFA) need

NOTES:

Results:

Normal: 7.1 – 7.4

Clinical implications

ALKALINE SALIVA

Clinical Implication	Additional information
Metabolic Acidosis	The body responds to an acidosis by causing an increase in respiration to blow off CO_2 and thus lower carbonic acid in the body, which leads to a more alkaline salivary pH.
Respiratory alkalosis	Situation of extreme physiological stress can cause respiratory alkalosis. Too much CO_2 is "blown off" from increased respirations or hyperventilation. This causes alkaline saliva.
Maldigestion	The more alkaline the saliva gets, the weaker the digestive juices in the stomach may become, causing maldigestion
Hypochlorhydria	Alkaline saliva may be another marker for hypochlorhydria, which can upset the gastrointestinal equilibrium causing dysbiosis, yeast etc. that thrive in an abnormal digestive pH.
Sympathetic dominance	Sympathetic dominance causes an increase excretion of potassium, which occurs with increased cellular acidity.
Dental tartar	Alkaline saliva is one of the major causes of tartar build-up on the teeth.

ACIDIC SALIVA

Clinical Implication	Additional information
Metabolic Alkalosis	The body responds to an alkalosis by causing a compensatory suppression of the respiratory center in an attempt to retain CO_2, which leads to increased levels of carbonic acid, and an acid saliva.
Respiratory acidosis	Respiratory acidosis is due to insufficient respirations or air exchange, which causes increased CO_2 in the blood and a concomitant acidic saliva.
Carbohydrate maldigestion	Effective carbohydrate digestion relies on the activation of alpha amylase in the saliva. A salivary pH below 7.1 will not provide the optimum pH for alpha amylase activity.
Pancreatic insufficiency	Improper digestion due to lack of enzymes can lead to an increase in metabolic acids which will cause acidity to build up in the interstitial fluids thus affecting salivary pH
Essential fatty acid deficiency	A salivary pH below 7.2 may indicate a deficiency in essential fatty acids.
Fat digestion problems	Excess dietary fats or an inability to completely metabolize fats will cause an increase in ketones, which will increase the acids present in the interstitium.
Dental caries	Acidic saliva is a leading cause of dental caries & tooth decay.

NOTES:

Interpreting Acid-Alkaline Imbalances from Take-Home Tests

The following table can be used to make the determination of whether or not an acid-alkaline imbalance exists in your patients:

Take-Home Test	Resp. Acid.	Met. Acid.	Resp. Alk.	Met. Alk.
Breath hold time (40 – 65)	**< 40**	**< 40**	**>65**	**> 65**
Respiration Rate (14 – 18)	**> 19 or < 13**	**> 19**	**> 19 or < 13**	**< 13**
Urine pH (6.4 – 6.8)	**< 6.4**	**<6.4**	**>6.8**	**>6.8**
Salivary pH (7.1 – 7.4)	**< 7.1**	**>7.4**	**>7.4**	**<7.1**

Note: In order to have a pH imbalance you must observe an imbalance in both the breath holding time and respiration rate, and have either or both the urine pH and salivary pH out of balance.

Clinical Findings In Patterns Of Acidosis And Alkalosis

PATTERN	METABOLIC ACIDOSIS	METABOLIC ALKALOSIS
Discussion	**A build-up of H+ in cellular fluids that leads to systemic acidosis**	**↑ Excretion of H+ or retention of HCO_3^- →systemic alkalosis**
Respiration rate	**Increased** The respiratory system compensates by ↑ the rate and depth of respiration to blow off CO_2 and ↓ carbonic acid levels	**Decreased** Suppression of respiratory centers causes ↓ rate and depth of respiration to retain CO_2 and ↑ carbonic acid levels
Breath hold time	**Decreased** Acidosis causes a ↓ O_2 transport and uptake leading to a ↓ ability to hold one's breath	**Increased** Alkalosis causes an ↑ O_2 transport and uptake leading to a ↑ ability to hold one's breath
Urine pH	**Decreased** **Acidic urine-** kidneys compensate by excreting H+ in urine and retaining bicarbonate	**Increased** **Alkaline urine-** Kidneys compensate by retaining H+ and excreting bicarbonate in urine
Saliva pH	**Increased** **Alkaline saliva-** ↑ respiratory rate lowers the dissolved carbonic acid levels resulting in alkaline saliva	**Decreased** **Acidic saliva-** ↓ respiratory rate increases dissolved carbonic acid levels resulting in acidic saliva

NOTES:

PATTERN	RESPIRATORY ACIDOSIS	RESPIRATORY ALKALOSIS
Discussion	**Retention of H+ due to ↓ excretion of CO_2 from lungs**	**Loss of H+ due to ↑ excretion of CO_2 from lungs- hyperventilation**
Respiration rate	**Decreased as a 1° cause** ↓ Respiration rate (hypoventilation) is the primary cause of acidosis in respiratory acidosis. **Increased in compensation** The respiration rate is ↑ in respiratory compensation for metabolic acidosis. Rate and depth of respiration is ↑ to blow off more CO_2 and ↓ carbonic acid levels.	**Increased as a 1° cause** ↑ Respiration rate (hyperventilation) is the primary cause of alkalosis in respiratory alkalosis **Decreased in compensation** The respiration rate is ↓ in respiratory compensation for metabolic alkalosis. Rate and depth of respiration is ↓ to retain more CO_2 and ↑ carbonic acid levels.
Breath hold time	**Decreased** Acidosis causes a ↓ O_2 transport and uptake leading to a ↓ ability to hold one's breath	**Increased** Alkalosis causes an ↑ O_2 transport and uptake leading to a ↑ ability to hold one's breath
Urine pH	**Decreased** **Acidic urine-** kidneys compensate by excreting H+ in urine and retaining bicarbonate	**Increased** **Alkaline urine-** Kidneys compensate by retaining H+ and excreting bicarbonate in urine
Saliva pH	**Decreased** **Acidic saliva-** ↑ levels of CO_2 and carbonic acid due to hypoventilation	**Increased** **Alkaline saliva-** ↓ levels of CO_2 & carbonic acid due to hyperventilation

NOTES:

Dr. Bieler's Salivary pH Acid Challenge

Background

Dr. Bieler's test is a dynamic measurement of the body's alkaline mineral reserves- one of the secondary buffering systems of the body. We are looking to see whether the body has the reserves necessary to respond to an acid challenge. During this test the body is challenged with an acid in the form of lemon juice. The initial acidity of the lemon juice will cause the saliva to buffer this acidity over the course of a few minutes by becoming more alkaline. We expect the saliva to get more alkaline to show that the body can respond to an acid challenge by marshalling up the necessary alkaline mineral reserves. If there are enough alkaline minerals in the body, the body will use them as a buffer. If there is an alkaline mineral insufficiency, the body may start to use ammonia as a buffer, which is an indication of low mineral reserves.

This test also allows us to see how stress and sympathetic dominance impact minerals reserves in the body. Increasing levels of stress to the point of adrenal exhaustion will cause the loss of the primary mineral reserves, which are composed of the alkaline minerals potassium, magnesium, sodium and calcium. In ideal situations the kidneys use these alkaline reserves to buffer metabolic acids that come through the tubules. In times of mineral insufficiency and stress, the body will resort to using ammonia, which combines with acid and is secreted in the urine as ammonium salts. The ammonia buffering system is used in cases when there is a deficiency in the alkaline minerals. In these situations the urine may have a strong ammonia smell.

The buffering activity measured in this test occurs in the mouth, salivary ducts and saliva. It is a measure of short term buffering, using the secondary buffering systems and does not rely on stomach absorption of the lemon juice for its effect.

Discussion

The alkaline mineral reserves get taken up into the lymphatic fluid, where they are used as a buffer for extracellular acids. The saliva, as a measure of lymph fluid, is the ideal place to measure such activity.

Supplies you will need to give patients

1. A copy of the handout "Dr. Bieler's Salivary pH Acid Challenge" (see handouts section in back of book).
2. 1 roll of pH paper
3. Inform them they will need to purchase lemon juice

Directions

1. The patient will use the pH test paper for this test. They should cut seven 2" strips of pH paper and lay out on paper towel.
2. Prepare lemon juice drink: 1 tablespoon of lemon juice and 1 tablespoon of water
3. Have patient make a pool of saliva in mouth and dip half of the strip, remove and measure pH. Record as baseline.

NOTES:

ABO Blood Typing

Background

ABO blood typing is a system of classifying blood according to differences in the antigenic make-up of red blood cells. Blood group typing is essential for a safe blood transfusion and is useful to apply this information for categorized typologies regarding diet and lifestyle variations as presented by Dr. James D'Adamo.

Discussion

 There are essentially two main types of marker proteins or antigens on the surface of RBC's. About 400 other antigens have been identified but since these various antigens are widely scattered throughout the population, these rarely cause transfusion problems and are cross matched prior to the procedure.

- The two main groups are classified as type A and type B. According to whether or not the person's blood contains one or the other, both, or neither, it is classified as A, B, AB, or O.

- The most common blood group is O, followed by A, then B, and finally AB. The precise frequency of each group differs among races.

- Blood group compatibilities depend on anti-A or anti-B antibodies present which react with the protein markers.

- As such, type O persons make universal donors as they posses neither antigen.

- Likewise, type AB individuals make universal recipients because they contain both antigens and do not form antibodies to either one.

Rh Factor

Another blood group system is the Rhesus factor (Rh factor). This system involves several antigens, the most important of which is factor D which is found in approximately 85% of the population labeled as Rh positive. The other 15% lack the factor and are considered Rh negative. The main importance of this test is in pregnancy of Rh-negative women. If the baby is Rh-positive, the mother may likely form antibodies against the baby's blood (Hemolytic dz of the newborn). Rh-negative women are given antibodies directed against factor D after delivery to prevent the development of anti-D antibodies in the mother, which would cause hemolytic disease in an Rh-positive infant. Transfusion of Rh-positive blood into an Rh-negative patient can also cause a serious reaction if the patient has had previous blood transfusions that contained the Rh antigen.

NOTES:

When would you ask your patient to run this test?

1. To identify their blood group and Rh factor
2. To help determine their appropriate blood typing diet

Supplies you will need to give patients

1. An Eldoncard for ABO blood typing available from Carolina Biologicals
2. Patient instructions that come with the Eldoncard

Directions

We recommend using the Eldoncard system to ascertain your patient's blood type. This is a procedure that can be done in the office or just as easily sent home with the patient. Each Eldoncard kit comes with the necessary equipment (sterile lancet, Eldoncard, and plastic comb for applying the blood to the cards) and instruction form to safely, reliably and quickly determine ABO blood type in 3 minutes. No special lab facilities are required. Each kit has a shelf life of 2 years, and after use the cards serve as documentation for an unlimited time.

1. Open the foil packet and remove the Eldoncard. You will notice that there are four squares on the card. Drop one full drop of tap water on to the reagent in each test panel. Do not use distilled water or saline.

2. Prepare the finger for blood collection:
   a. Run finger under hot water for 1 minute to get blood into the finger.
   b. Dry finger with clean cloth.
   c. Hold finger firmly and quickly and smoothly pierce the skin with the sterile lancet.
   d. Gently "milk" the hand and finger to get a drop of blood on the finger tip.

3. Touch the blood drop from below with the four teeth of the plastic comb, so that a drop of blood settles on the end of each tooth.

4. You will now have drops of blood on each of the four teeth of the plastic comb.

5. Rub the blood from the four teeth onto the four squares of the eldoncard. Rub quickly to and fro for 30 seconds. Spread the blood right out to all sides of the panels.

6. Wait 1 minute, and in the interim record your name and other data in the space provided on the card.

7. Tilt the card back and forth and from side to side for 2 minutes.

8. Read and record the results. See the chart on the following page for interpretation)

9. In order to be certain of the appearance of the negative reactions, it is recommended to tilt the card once more two minutes after the reading.

NOTES:

Note: The dry card may be preserved with plastic for your records

Results

The following is an interpretation chart that accompanies the Eldoncards.

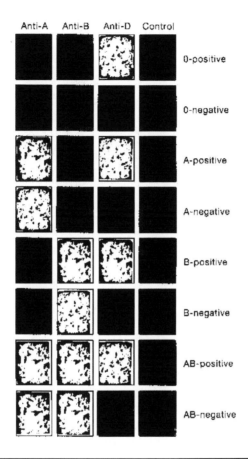

ABO Blood Typing and Diet

The connection between diet and blood typing has been pioneered by Dr. Peter D'Adamo, Naturopathic physician. Over the last 30 years he has been using the ABO blood typing system to determine which type of diet is most compatible with the individual.

Importance of knowing your blood type

The reason blood grouping is important in determining a person's diet is due to molecules called lectins which are found in foods. A large majority of lectins are destroyed by cooking but a small amount will survive the cooking process to make it into your digestive tract. If the digestive process in the stomach (hydrochloric acid and pepsin) or upper small intestine (digestive enzymes) is in anyway compromised the lectins can pass undigested into the lower small intestine, where the immune tissue will recognize these lectins as either being self or non-self. If raw foods are eaten, a greater

NOTES:

percentage of lectins will pass into the intestinal lumen. If the digestive processes are intact i.e. adequate amounts of HCl and digestive enzymes, this should pose no increased risk.

The immune reaction to lectins is dependent upon the ABO blood type. If the lectin is perceived as non-self the immune system will mount a non-specific immune reaction, causing the release of histamine, complement activation and mucosal secretory IgA release. This will cause mild intestinal inflammation. Prolonged inflammation in the intestines can lead to increased intestinal hyperpermeability (Leaky Gut Syndrome), and the break down of the intestinal brush border. The hyperpermeability and diminished absorptive surface area allows for almost free movement of large macromolecules into the portal circulation and lymph vessels, setting up eventual antibody formation. The person is now at high risk for the development of other diseases.

Each blood type reacts to a specific group of dietary lectins. We recommend reading Dr. D'Adamo's book, Eat Right for your Type to get more information on how to use the ABO blood type to determine the right diet for your patient.

Get master copies of all of the handouts in the Take-Home Testing book. Visit:
www.BloodChemistryAnalysis.com

Clinical implications

Result	Clinical Implication
Blood Type O	Blood type O is the oldest blood type and appeared and was the prevalent type among hunter-gatherers. They typically had a high protein, high meat diet. Because of this group O individuals tend to secrete higher amounts of stomach acid in order to digest the protein. Blood type O individuals will typically have a greater incidence of gastric ulcer disease than the other blood groups. Blood group O is about 46% of the American population.
Blood Type A	The next blood group to evolve was the blood group A, which evolved in response to increasing agrarian practices. Type A blood types evolved very quickly as a response to increasingly dense population centers. People with type A blood tend to be more resistant to infection. Blood group A individuals will secrete less stomach acid than type Os, and do best with vegetarian food sources. Protein requirements are not any less than a group O person but the source is typically from vegetables and legumes. Type A people tend to have greater levels of heart disease, cancer, and diabetes. Group A comprises 42% of the American population.

NOTES:

Blood Type B	Blood group B evolved in cultures that consumed higher quantities of dairy products. This group tends to function better and is associated with cultures which use higher amounts of fermented dairy products. These people tend to function better on diets which are high in dairy products and fish. Group B persons tend to have higher incidences of urinary tract diseases, such as kidney and bladder infections. Group B persons make up about 7% of the American population.
Blood Type AB	Blood group AB was the last to evolve. Nicknamed the "modern group" by Dr. D'Adamo this blood type has evolved to tolerate a wide range of foods. The diet that suits the AB blood type best combines the characteristics of groups A & B. They can tolerate small amounts of many different foods which would be reactive in the other blood groups. They can tolerate a diet higher in seafood, some dairy, nuts and grains. Blood group AB comprises 4% of the American population.

Interfering Factors:

There is a very small chance of false negatives or positives if the procedure outlined above is followed according to the instructions.

NOTES:

Pulse Challenge Food Sensitivity Testing

Background

There are many different methods for assessing food allergies and sensitivities. Each has its own advantages and disadvantages. The pulse challenge food sensitivity testing method was developed by Dr. Arthur Coca over 40 years ago. Arthur Coca, MD was one of the pre-eminent allergists in the U.S. He was honorary president of the American Association of Immunologists. Founder and first editor of the *Journal of Immunology*, one of the foremost medical publications in this field, and taught at Cornell, University of Pennsylvania, and Post-graduate studies at Columbia University.

His method of allergy/intolerance assessment called The Coca Pulse Testing method is simple and extremely effective at identifying foods that a patient may be intolerant, allergic or sensitive to.

Discussion

 This is a simple yet extremely effective way to identify foods to which a patient may be allergic, intolerant or sensitive. The test is based on the fact that stress from an allergic food will cause the pulse to increase.

- Foods to which you are intolerant are stressful and will reveal themselves by speeding up your pulse. Laboratory tests which are often less accurate than this method could easily cost over a thousand dollars.

- Using this method Dr. Coca was able to eliminate a host of symptoms and conditions simply by identifying and eliminating food from the diet to which a patient was intolerant.

- The advantage of this method is that the patient can do much of the assessment at home.

- As health recovery proceeds, some foods to which your patient has a sensitivity may be reintroduced in moderation using the pulse to monitor their acceptability.

- Understanding and using the test as a tool can help you to help your patients to be free from the ill effects of eating foods that are not right for them.

How does the Pulse Challenge work?

- The sensory information from the taste buds in the mouth informs the CNS as to the nature of the test substance.
- If the test substance is stressful to the body, there will be a brief reaction that causes the heart to beat faster.

When would you ask your patient to run this test?

1. To help your patients find out the foods they are intolerant to.

2. To help find the environmental toxins your patients are sensitive to.

NOTES:

Supplies you will need to give patients

1. A copy of the handouts "Diet/Pulse Record", "Pulse Testing Individual Foods", and "Pulse Test Record" (see handouts section in back of book).

Directions

The Pulse Challenge Food Sensitivity Testing incorporates two methods of assessing food sensitivities.

1. The initial pulse testing procedure uses a handout called **Diet/Pulse Record** (see handouts section in back of book). This initial pulse testing procedure is designed to identify meals that may or may not include foods that your patients may be allergic, intolerant or sensitive to. This technique can be used along side a diet diary.

2. The second pulse testing procedure is designed to identify individual foods that your patients are sensitive to. This procedure uses a handout called **Pulse Testing Individual Foods** (see handouts section in back of book). Using this handout your patients can perform a simple 2 minute self-test to determine if a particular food causes a stressful reaction. The patient can either choose their own foods to test, or you can write in the foods that you suspect they are sensitive to, and write those on the form. The Pulse testing method is also sensitive to supplements, and can be used to determine whether or not a particular supplement is causing stress to the system. Many doctors use this technique to make sure that their prescriptions are not causing stress to their patients.

Diet/Pulse Record

1. Your patient will take their pulse 14 times across three days.
   a. Once before getting out of bed
   b. Before each meal
   c. Three times after each meal, and finally
   d. Before bed
2. They should record what foods were in the meals and also feelings, activities and cravings across the day.
3. For best results they should avoid snacks between meals. If they eat a snack they should write it down.
4. For accuracy they should take a full one-minute pulse.
5. They should avoid smoking for the three-day test, which will change test results.
6. Once they have completed the tracking form they should bring the results in for assessment.
7. By the end of three days you should have enough data to begin the next stage- using pulse testing to find individual foods.

Pulse testing Individual Foods

1. The patient should get into a relaxed place, sit down and take a deep breath.
2. They should establish their baseline pulse by counting for one full minute.

NOTES:

3. They should then place a sample of food in their mouth (on their tongue). They should refrain from swallowing. They will need to taste it for approximately one-half minute.

4. It is important to test only one food at a time. Testing individual ingredients will yield specific information, compared with testing foods containing multiple ingredients. Testing a banana, for example, yields more specific and therefore more valuable information than testing banana bread.

5. The patient should retake their pulse while the food remains in their mouth and write down their "after" pulse on the pulse test record form.

6. They should discard the tested ingredient, rather than swallowing it.

7. If a reaction occurred, they should rinse their mouth out with some purified water and spit the water out.

8. Wait two minutes, then they should retest the pulse to see if it has returned to its baseline. If it hasn't, they should wait a couple of minutes more and retest.

9. They should continue to retest until the pulse has returned to normal.

10. Once the pulse has returned to its normal rate they can test the next food.

11. They can repeat the procedure as frequently as they like, as long they let the pulse return to its baseline before testing the next food.

Diet/Pulse Record 3-day test interpretation

Result	Interpretation
Pulse greater standing than sitting	This is a positive sign of food or environmental sensitivities.
Daily maximal pulse rate varies more than two beats i.e. Monday 72, Tuesday 78, Wednesday 76	This is a strong sign of sensitivities
A minimum pulse-rate that does not regularly occur "before rising" but at some other time of day.	This is a sign of sensitivity to dust, dust mites or something in the sleeping environment.

NOTES:

A 6 – 8 point or more increase after a meal	This is a sure sign that you were sensitive to something during that meal.
A 6 – 8 point or more increase 30 minutes after a meal	This is an indication that there is a sensitivity to something that is quickly absorbed i.e. refined carbohydrates.
A 6 – 8 point or more increase 60 minutes after a meal	This is an indication that there is a sensitivity to complex carbohydrates in that meal.
A 6 – 8 point or more increase 90 minutes after a meal	This is an indication that there is a sensitivity to proteins in that meal.
Pulse rate is constant for three days in a row	You can be pretty sure that all "food sensitivities" have been avoided on those days.
Ingestion of a frequently eaten food causes no acceleration of the pulse	One can be fairly certain that your patient was not allergic or sensitive to any food in that meal.

NOTES:

Patient Handouts

NOTES:

HCl Challenge Test

Purpose: This Test is useful for assessing the integrity of the stomach lining and the amount of supplemental HCl (stomach acid) that is compatible with good health. There is a correlation between a strong showing on this test and a strong digestive function (i.e. acid and enzyme production).

Meal 1: Take 1 capsule of supplemental HCl at the **beginning**, after the first few bites of a substantial complex meal (i.e. on that contains protein). Do not test a small meal or one that consists of only fruit, a light salad or a simple bowl of cereal. Stop if you experience any stomach irritation. (see below)

Meal 2: Take 2 capsules at the **beginning** of the next complex meal.

Meal 3: Take 3 capsules at the **beginning** of the next complex meal and so on with successive meals until you reach 4 capsules.

STOP taking the supplemental HCl if and when you react and have the following symptoms:
1. Feeling of warmth or pressure in your stomach
2. Irritation i.e. heartburn, stomach ache

If you experience the above reaction drink a tall glass of water to quench the reaction. You may take and antacid i.e. Tums, Alka-Seltzer Gold, or baking soda and water – ½ tsp. per cup, if it is necessary to neutralize the acidity.

Name:_____	**Date:**_____
_____ **Capsules caused a reaction.**	
Describe:_____	
_____	

Caution: This test is contraindicated in individuals with a current or past history of ulcers, as well as those who are currently taking antacids or acid blocking medications.

Please fax this back to the office or drop it by the office.

NOTES:

Bowel Transit Time
Instruction for Self-Testing

Name:_____ Date:_____

The Bowel Transit Time is an excellent test to measure how long it takes for a substance to be eliminated through the bowel. Optimally it should take between 18 to 24 hours for food to completely move through your digestive tract. This indicates that you are probably breaking down and absorbing well. This test uses charcoal, an inert substance, to measure the transit time. Charcoal will stain your stool black or gray, and thus provides a conveniently visible medium for measuring the transit time.

Instructions:

1. Swallow 4 charcoal capsules at the evening meal. Record the date and time you swallowed the capsules under "Time In" on the form below.
2. After every bowel movement, observe the stool under bright light. When you see a black or charcoal gray stool record the date and time under "Time Color First Appears" on the form below.
3. Calculate the number of hours between the time noted under "Time in" and the time noted under "Time Color First Appears" and write this time (in hours) in the form below. This is the time it took for the charcoal to pass through the digestive tract.
4. Continue to examine every stool and note the time and date when the color has completely disappeared.
5. Wait five (5) days to allow the marker to clear fully from the intestines and then repeat this process again, following the same instructions.

	Time and Date In	Time Color first appears	Transit time (hours)	Time completely cleared
# 1				
# 2				

Please indicate on the form below if any of the following are noticed in your stool:

☐ Blood on the stool	☐ Undigested food in stool	☐ Mucous on stool
☐ Stool is loose	☐ Stool is hard	☐ Stool is floating
☐ Ribbon like stool	☐ Large caliber stool	☐ Small, round and hard
☐ Brown colored	☐ Dark brown colored	☐ Yellow
☐ Black	☐ Tan or clay colored	☐ Offensive odor

NOTES:

Directions for Measuring Blood Glucose.

1. Wash your hands. Invisible material on the fingers can cause erroneous readings.
2. Do not wipe fingers with alcohol. This only dries the finger out and can cause calluses. It is highly unlikely that you will get a finger infection by not using alcohol.
3. Rinse the fingers under warm water unless the fingers are already warm. Blood flow increases when the fingers are warm.
4. Sort out the supplies for measuring blood glucose: finger-stick device loaded with a sterile lancet, the glucometer, test strips, and tissue for blotting the blood.
5. Insert a fresh strip into the glucometer. Follow the directions for loading the test strips into your particular unit.
6. The spring loaded finger-stick device is used to obtain a drop of blood. The pressure of the device on the finger determines how deep the lancet will puncture the skin. It should be deep enough to get an adequate amount of blood, but not so deep as to cause bruising or pain.
7. Contrary to popular opinion one of the best areas for getting a blood sample is the back of the hand. Prick the fingers near the nails, or between the first and second joints. The advantages of using these areas are less pain and more chance of getting an adequate drop of blood. You will also prevent calluses by repeatedly using the fleshy pads on the finger tips. By all means use these areas too if the thought of pricking the back of hand is off-putting.
8. Cock the spring-loaded finger stick device and prick any finger. Squeeze the finger using a pumping action rather than constant pressure. You should aim to get a drop of blood about 1/16th of an inch in diameter.
9. Touch the blood to the test strip.
10. The glucometer will start a count down procedure once the blood has been absorbed by the test strip. After the countdown has started inspect the drop of blood to see that the test strip has been properly covered by the blood drop. If not discard the strip and begin the process over again. It is essential that the strip be covered in blood to prevent erroneous readings.
11. If you are the only person using the glucometer it is not necessary to use a fresh lancet every time. If others are using the unit, please remove the used lancet to prevent possible contamination for future users.
12. The whole process from start to finish should take approximately 2 minutes.
13. Record the number from the glucometer on your form.

NOTES:

Take-Home Testing Patient Handouts- **Blood Sugar Tracking Form**

Blood Sugar Tracking Form

DAY & TIME		BLOOD TEST RESULTS								COMMENTS
		BREAKFAST		LUNCH		DINNER		BED TIME	UPON WAKING	Weight change, diet or mealtime changes, illness, stress, changes in activity etc.
		Before	1 hour After	Before	1 hour After	Before	1 hour After			
SUN	TIME									
	RESULT									
MON	TIME									
	RESULT									
TUE	TIME									
	RESULT									
WED	TIME									
	RESULT									

NOTES:

Take-Home Testing Patient Handouts- **Blood Sugar Tracking Form**

DAY & TIME		BLOOD TEST RESULTS								COMMENTS Weight change, diet or mealtime changes, illness, stress, changes in activity etc.
		BREAKFAST		LUNCH		DINNER		BED TIME	UPON WAKING	
		Before	1 hour After	Before	1 hour After	Before	1 hour After			
THU	TIME									
	RESULT									
FRI	TIME									
	RESULT									
SAT	TIME									
	RESULT									

COMMENTS: _____

_____

_____

_____

_____

_____

56

NOTES:

Zinc Taste Test and Zinc Challenge

Name:_____ Date:_____

The Zinc Taste Test is an excellent test for assessing zinc deficiency. The zinc challenge will help us determine how zinc deficient you are and what type of therapy you may need. Zinc is one of the most important trace minerals. It is essential for tissue growth, skin integrity, immunity, blood sugar control, and essential fatty acid regulation. Unfortunately, zinc deficiency is widespread and can lead to a number of problems including infertility and lowered immunity. The zinc taste test is an easy method of assessing your zinc levels.

Instructions:
1. Make sure your mouth is free of strong tastes, such as mint. Have a stopwatch, timer, or watch with a second hand on it, because you will be timing how soon you taste the Zinc Taste Test solution.
2. Measure out 1 tablespoon of the Aqueous Zinc (the Zinc Taste Test solution), put it into your mouth, hold and swish around your mouth, but do not swallow.
3. Start timing as soon as the solution is in your mouth and note when you first taste the solution.
4. Swallow after 30 seconds.
5. On the form below note the time it took to first taste the solution and describe the strength of taste or presence of an after taste in the column marked **Initial test**.

	Time to taste solution	Describe Strength of Taste or After-Taste			
Initial Test		☐ Immediate taste. Strong metallic.	☐ Not so strong taste. Delayed metallic	☐ No taste noted initially. Sweet or bitter.	☐ Tasteless or tastes like water.
		No Need for Further testing		**Move on to the Zinc Challenge test**	

Zinc Challenge
The Zinc Challenge is used to assess how zinc deficient you may be.

Directions
1. Follow the same directions for doing the Zinc Taste Test.
2. Repeat the test successively, resting 30 seconds between tests.
3. Note on the form below the time it took to taste the solution, and the strength of taste.
4. Repeat this process until you have a strong immediate taste, or you perform 6 successive tests with no taste noted. At this point discontinue the testing.

NOTES:

IODINE PATCH TEST

Name:_____ Date:_____

The Iodine Patch Test is an excellent test for assessing for iodine deficiency. Despite the fortification of our salt and food with iodine many people are iodine deficient. Iodine is essential for the proper synthesis of thyroid hormone in the body. Unfortunately iodine deficiency is widespread because of the prevalence of chemicals such as chlorine, bromine and fluoride in our environment and water supply. These chemicals will quickly deplete iodine from the body and interfere with iodine metabolism leading to a number of problems including hypothyroidism, lowered vitality, cognitive dysfunction, lowered immunity, and obesity. The iodine patch test is an easy method of assessing your iodine levels.

Instructions:

1. You will use the bottle of topical iodine supplied by your physician or in the test kit. Remember this is to be used topically and not orally.

2. Paint the skin of the inside of your forearm or abdomen with a 2 inch square patch of 2% iodine solution, being careful not to get the solution on your clothes as it will stain. Note the time you put the iodine onto the skin on the form below.

3. Air dry the patch before putting clothes on.

4. You will need to monitor how quickly the patch fades.

5. Avoid soaking in hot tubs or baths for 24 hours, as the chlorine or bromine in the water will cause the iodine to patch to come off.

6. Note on the form below how soon after application the iodine patch has disappeared.

Time Iodine Put on Skin	Time Color Disappears	# of hours it took to completely disappear

NOTES:

METABOLIC pH ASSESSMENT

Name:_____   Date:_____

It is essential that your body has a well balanced pH system. pH is the measurement of acidity and alkalinity in the body. Certain areas of the body require an acid environment to work optimally, e.g. your stomach, while others require an alkaline environment, e.g. the small intestine. Many systems of your body operate most effectively with a properly balanced pH. For instance, an optimal pH of the blood is needed for oxygen delivery to your cells and for the correct action of insulin to control blood sugar levels. The body uses a number of complex systems to keep the pH within a normal and optimal range, and the following series of tests are designed to see if those regulatory mechanisms are working properly.

The two main systems of regulation are the respiratory system and your kidneys, which work in concert to finely regulate the levels of acid and alkaline in your body. By measuring how long you can hold your breath, how many breaths you take in a minute, and your urine and salivary pH we can determine what areas of your body are in need of further support to bring your pH system into balance.

Instructions

1. Breath Hold Test

    a. This test is an actual measurement of how long you can hold a deep breath. You will need a stopwatch, a watch with a second hand or a timer to time the breath holding.

    b. It is hard to time one's own breath-hold time, so it is best to have a family member or friend do the timing.

    c. You should be seated and should take a deep breath and hold it as long as you can. You should stop when it begins to feel uncomfortable or you feel as if you need to take another breath. This is not meant to be a test of endurance!

    d. When you can no longer hold your breath, let it out, and record the number of seconds the breath was held on the chart below.

2. Respiration Rate

    a. This test is an actual measurement of how many breaths you take in a minute. This is your respiration rate. You will need a stopwatch, a watch with a second hand, or a timer to time your respiration rate.

    b. It is hard to time one's respiration rate because you will most likely alter your respiration rate if you are doing the timing, so it is best to have a family member or friend do the timing.

    c. You should be lying down when this test is performed and the trick is to breath as normally and unconsciously as possible.

NOTES:

PULSE TESTING INDIVIDUAL FOODS

Name:_____ Date:_____

A simple 2 ½ minute self-test to determine if a particular food or supplement causes a stressful reaction.

Instructions:

1. Sit down, take a deep breath, and relax.
2. Establish your baseline pulse by counting your heart beat for a full minute and record your pulse in the "Before" space in the Pulse Test Record below.
3. Put a sample of a food or supplement to evaluate in your mouth (on your tongue). You may chew but refrain from swallowing. However, you do need to taste it for approximately one-half minute.
4. Retake your pulse (the food or the supplement remains in your mouth). Write down your "After" pulse on the Pulse Test Record below.
5. Discard the tested ingredient (do not swallow) and repeat the procedure to test other foods or supplements. Repeat the procedure as frequently as you like, as long as you always return to your normal pulse before testing the next food.
6. Fax this form to our office or bring this record with you to your next appointment.

PULSE TEST RECORD

Food	Pulse Before/After	Difference	Food	Pulse Before/After	Difference
	____/____			____/____	
	____/____			____/____	
	____/____			____/____	
	____/____			____/____	
	____/____			____/____	
	____/____			____/____	
	____/____			____/____	
	____/____			____/____	
	____/____			____/____	
	____/____			____/____	

NOTES:

The "Four Quadrants of Functional Diagnosis" Diagnostic Education for the *Functional Age*

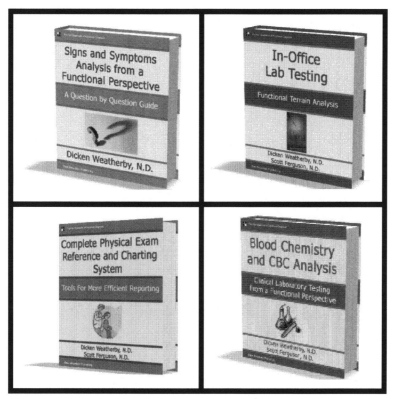

Most of us at some point or other have come to recognize that the diagnostic tests we learned in medical school taught us nothing about how to uncover our patients' functional problems. This is why I wrote my first book, *"Blood Chemistry and CBC Analysis- Clinical Laboratory Testing From a Functional Perspective"* with my colleague Dr. Scott Ferguson, to make the wealth of functional information you can get from a standard Chemistry Screen and CBC available to health care practitioners. This book and other products in my "Four Quadrants of Functional Diagnosis" series are designed to give you and your practice the same functional diagnostic education that thousands of practitioners have been using successfully in their practices.

The *Four Quadrants of Functional Diagnosis* will help you:
- Get excellent patient results
- Dramatically improve your clinical outcomes
- Get more referrals
- Cut the amount of time you spend analyzing your patient cases
- Set up a system of functional tests that will be the envy of all your colleagues

In preparing for the Functional Age, the rules on how to manage the diagnostic information in your practice have changed. You can no longer blindly use the same tests every one else is using and hope to get different results. The Functional Age will require that you have more information to be able to properly find the cause of your patients' problems. *Signs and Symptoms Analysis from A Functional Perspective, Boost Clinic Income With an In-Office Lab System,* and *The Functional Blood Chemistry Analysis System* were developed for practitioners just like you who recognize the need for a new paradigm in diagnostic information. Practitioners who realize that the Pathological Age is over and the Functional Age has begun.

Dr. Dicken Weatherby, Naturopathic Physician

Functional Blood Chemistry Analysis

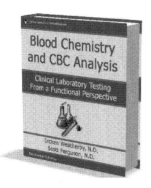

Blood Chemistry and CBC Analysis- Clinical Laboratory Testing from a Functional Perspective

This book presents a diagnostic system of blood chemistry and CBC analysis that focuses on physiological function as a marker of health. By looking for optimum function we increase our ability to detect dysfunction long before disease manifests. Conventional lab testing becomes a truly preventative and prognostic tool. A must for any practitioners who wants to get more from the tests they are already running.
Printed Book $65.00 (in the U.S.A.) ISBN: 0-9761367-1-6

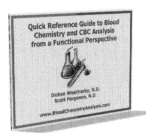

Quick Reference Guide to Blood Chemistry Analysis From a Functional Perspective

This guide is the perfect companion to our Blood Chemistry and CBC Analysis Book. It is a complete reference for interpreting, analyzing, and finding the underlying cause of your patients' functional complaints. You will find yourself referring to this guide over and over again.
Printed Book $35.00 (in the U.S.A.) ISBN: 0-9761367-8-3

Blood Chemistry University - Functional Blood Chemistry Analysis Online Training

The Functional Blood Chemistry Analysis Training Program at Blood Chemistry University is a complete road map to success that shows you exactly how to approach each blood chemistry analysis step by step. This online training includes 12 training modules that show you how to get the most out of your blood chemistry tests.

A functional diagnosis of your patients' blood test results is one of the most effective diagnostic tools to get to the bottom of the myriad of health complaints your patients present with. Gain expert status, and increase business by being the one doctor who can tell patients exactly what their blood tests mean. **http://www.BloodChemistryTraining.com**

Other Functional Diagnostic Tools

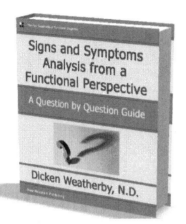

Signs and Symptoms Analysis From a Functional Perspective

This book takes a critical look at the myriad of signs and symptoms a patient presents with. Using a comprehensive signs and symptoms questionnaire you can look at the symptom burden in specific systems of the body, address some of the more obscure symptoms, and track changes over time. Organized by body systems, this book provides the nutritional and functional explanations behind the 322 questions on Dr. Weatherby's 4-page questionnaire.

Printed Book $65.00 (in the U.S.A.) ISBN: 0-9761367-2-4

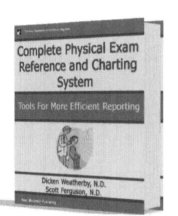

Complete PE Reference and Charting System

Drs. Weatherby and Ferguson have put together report forms for all the major physical examinations commonly performed in your office (i.e. cardiovascular, lung, abdominal, neurological examinations). These report forms provide an easy method of charting and filing your physical examination results.

The accompanying reference cards fit neatly into your white coat and provide a detailed explanation of all the tests on each report form and are an excellent "exam-side" reference to refresh your memory on all the different tests that make up each examination.

Printed Reference Cards and CD $65.00 (in the U.S.A.)

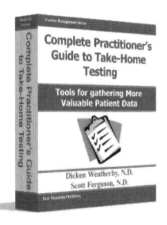

Complete Practitioner's Guide to Take-Home Testing

Drs. Weatherby and Ferguson have put together a series of 17 take-home tests that you can give to your patients to perform in between their office visits. These tests will allow you to assess for digestion, elimination, zinc status, pH regulation, hypothyroid conditions, iodine insufficiency, blood type, and food and other sensitivities and intolerances. Patient "homework" is an important method of gathering patient data and encouraging compliance.

Printed Book $45.00 (in the U.S.A.) ISBN: 0-9761367-7-5

To Order Any Functional Diagnostic Product Please Visit Our Website
www.BloodChemistryAnalysis.com

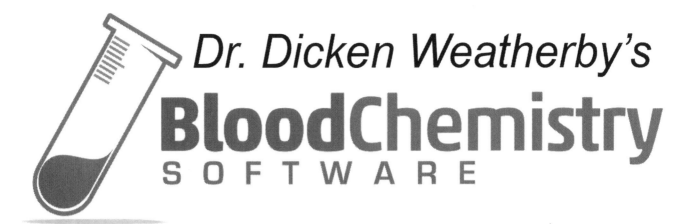
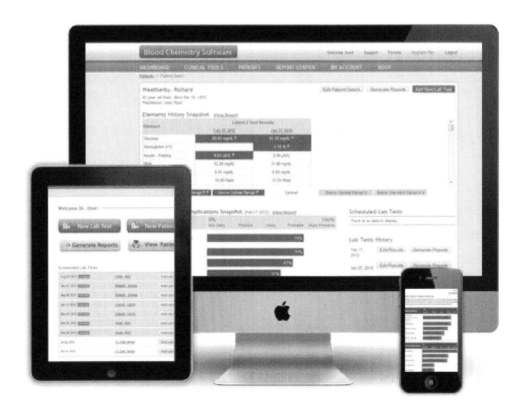

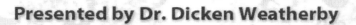

Blood Chemistry University™

Presented by Dr. Dicken Weatherby

Blood Chemistry University Provides You With Everything You'll Need to Be Successful........

 12 "Look Over Dicken's Shoulder" Online Video Training Sessions

 Lifetime Access to "Blood Chemistry University"

 Audio MP3 and PDF Downloads From All Sessions!

 8 Hours of Bonus Training From FM Experts

4 Things You Will Know After You Join Blood Chemistry University:

✓ An understanding of the implications for blood tests that are outside the normal value and implications of blood tests that fall outside of an optimal range.

✓ A knowledge of what tests to order....You will learn what tests deserve to be on your standard panel, and what tests don't.

✓ How to turn your regular blood chemistry and CBC/Hematology test into an incredible prognostic marker for dysfunction.

✓ How to put it all together....You will have an understanding of the patterns that exist between tests and the likely dysfunctions associated with the patterns.

Dr. Weatherby's "Functional Blood Chemistry Analysis System"....What Every Health Care Practitioner Ought to Be Using In *THEIR* Functional Medicine Practices!!!"

➡ Do you want exciting new diagnostic skills to get your patients and your practice to the next level of success?

➡ Do you like rapid results and excellent clinical outcomes?

➡ Are you are looking for new tools and techniques to dramatically improve your clinical outcomes?

➡ Do you want more referrals?

➡ Do you want to take on those hard to treat cases no one else can work with?

How would you like to learn everything you need to know about the functional analysis of your patients' blood tests which will:

✓ Put you on the cutting edge of preventative diagnosis.

✓ Help you get more from the tests you are already performing.

✓ Hone your blood chemistry analysis skills.

✓ Show you how these tests can be used as a prognostic marker for dysfunction.

✓ Cut the amount of time you spend analyzing your patient's blood tests.

http://BloodChemistryTraining.com

Printed in Great Britain
by Amazon